HIV/AIDS
and HIV/AIDS-Related
Terminology
A Means of Organizing
the Body of Knowledge

HIV/AIDS
and HIV/AIDS–Related
Terminology
A Means of Organizing the Body of Knowledge

Jeffrey T. Huber, PhD
Mary L. Gillaspy, MS, MLS

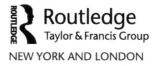

Routledge
Taylor & Francis Group

NEW YORK AND LONDON

First published 1996 by

The Haworth Press, Inc., 10 Alice Street, Binghamton, NY 13904-1580

This edition published 2013 by Routledge

Routledge
Taylor & Francis Group
711 Third Avenue,
New York, NY 10017, USA

Routledge
Taylor & Francis Group
2 Park Square, Milton Park,
Abingdon, Oxfordshire OX14 4RN

First issued in paperback 2016

Routledge is an imprint of the Taylor & Francis Group, an informa business

Library of Congress Cataloging-in-Publication Data

Huber, Jeffrey T.
    HIV/AIDS and HIV/AIDS-related terminology : a means of organizing the body of knowledge / Jeffrey T. Huber, Mary L. Gillaspy.
        p.   cm.
    Includes bibliographical references and index.
    ISBN 1-56024-970-6 (alk. paper)
    1. AIDS (Disease)–Terminology. 2. HIV infections–Terminology. 3. Subject headings–HIV infections. 4. Subject headings–AIDS (Disease) I. Gillaspy, Mary L. II. Title.
RC607.A26H896   1996
616.97′92′0014–dc20   96-1981
                                                                                             CIP

ISBN 13: 978-1-138-97184-4 (pbk)
ISBN 13: 978-1-56024-970-2 (hbk)

This book is offered as a vehicle for managing the growing body of knowledge surrounding the complexities of HIV and AIDS. It is dedicated to all individuals affected by this pandemic.

ABOUT THE AUTHORS

Jeffrey T. Huber, PhD, is currently Research Information Scientist at Vanderbilt University in Nashville, Tennessee. Until recently, he was Assistant Professor at the School of Library and Information Studies at Texas Women's University in Denton, Texas, where he was also Co-Chair of the University's Task Force on HIV/AIDs. Dr. Huber is the author of a number of articles concerning AIDS information and is the editor of *How to Find Information About AIDS, Second Edition* and *Dictionary of AIDS-Related Terminology.* A member of the American Library Association, the Medical Library Association, and the International Society for AIDS Education, Dr. Huber has delivered many presentations at national conferences and meetings.

Mary L. Gillaspy, MS, MLS, is Manager of Health Education at M. D. Anderson Cancer Research Center in Houston, Texas. For fourteen years, she worked in a school district of Garden City, Kansas. While she was an English teacher for grades 9-12 during most of her time there, she also held positions as English as a Second Language Coordinator and as Coordinator for Student Services. In the latter capacity, she developed and implemented an AIDS education plan for school administrators, teachers, parents, and secondary school students. In 1987, she received the University of Chicago Outstanding Teacher Award. Ms. Gillaspy is a member of the American Library Association, the Medical Library Association, and the Special Libraries Association.

CONTENTS

Acknowledgments

Thanks are due to many people for helping to make this book a reality. Jean Hofacket, Director of Library Operations at the AIDS Information Network in Philadelphia, originally supported our use of her controlled vocabulary in our efforts to assert bibliographic control over the growing collection of materials at Dallas's AIDS Resource Center. Sheryl and Joe Kelly supplied the fourth edition of the *HIV/AIDS Curriculum* developed by the Mountain-Plains Regional AIDS Education and Training Center. Alan Hamill, DO, guided the development of the medical management section and provided valuable information regarding alternative therapies for HIV. Reverend James E. Liggett consulted on the development of the religious aspects section of the work. Leonard C. Bruno, Senior Science Specialist at the Library of Congress, assisted with the hierarchical arrangement of United States government agencies. Laura MacMurdy, MLS, reviewed the section on clinical manifestations of HIV and suggested portions of its ultimate arrangement.

Finally, special gratitude is reserved for Jamie Schield, the Director of Community Center Services and Education at the AIDS Resource Center in Dallas, Texas. Jamie's dream of adding a resource and information center to the many services provided by the agency was realized by mid-1995. His vision, support, encouragement, and unfailing optimism made development and testing of this work possible.

Introduction

HIV/AIDS and HIV/AIDS-Related Terminology: A Means of Organizing the Body of Knowledge has evolved from an effort to organize collections of information on the human immunodeficiency virus (HIV) and acquired immunodeficiency syndrome (AIDS). Existing systems, such as the Library of Congress Subject Headings (LCSH), Medical Subject Headings (MeSH), Sears, and those specific to HIV/AIDS, do not adequately represent the complex, cross-disciplinary nature of the disease. General works–ones not limited to HIV/AIDS (LCSH, MeSH, and Sears)–fail to represent the intricacies of the malady; while those that have been produced in response to the illness and its impact on various communities do not include specifics concerning biomedical aspects of HIV and associated diseases and infections. *HIV/AIDS and HIV/AIDS-Related Terminology: A Means of Organizing the Body of Knowledge* represents the multifaceted body of HIV/AIDS knowledge as it is reflected in such basic works as the following:

The AIDS Knowledge Base
Dictionary of AIDS Related Terminology
Textbook of AIDS Medicine
AIDS: Etiology, Diagnosis, Treatment and Prevention
AIDS Information Network
Educational Materials Database Thesaurus
HIV/AIDS Curriculum
Medical Subject Headings: Annotated Alphabetic List
Medical Subject Headings: Tree Structures

Medical Subject Headings, or MeSH, is the premier controlled vocabulary for medical and biomedical topics in the English language. Because of its importance and excellence in these areas, terms common to MeSH in this work are indicated with an asterisk (e.g., Chemistry*). When the term in this vocabulary is different from MeSH only in that it is presented in a singular or noninverted form, it is indicated with a "greater than" sign (e.g., Provirus >). These notations are made for two reasons: first, it indicates that the term is likely to be found often in the biomedical literature; and second, it leads people familiar with the MeSH tools to these resources, if further specificity is needed to provide access to a topic.

Even though some terms in this schema are common to MeSH, they do not necessarily have the same meaning. For example, the term *Practice guidelines** in MeSH is specifically used to denote works concerning guidelines as patient-care decision-support tools. *Practice guideline*, on the other hand, is used by indexers at the National Library of Medicine to indicate a publication type. In this schema, *Practice guidelines**, located under ~Publication Types, may be used either way. SEE references are provided from MeSH terms to preferred terms in this arrangement.

Yet another departure from MeSH is the use of single terms to refer not only to the diseases, syndromes, or conditions caused by an infectious agent but also to the infectious agent itself. For example, MeSH separates *Hantavirus** from *Hantavirus infections**; in this schema, the single term *Hantavirus** is used to refer to works concerning either of these topics.

This work is presented as a tool to facilitate the organization and management of the body of knowledge concerning infection due to HIV and its end stage, AIDS, and is intended to apply to works in all formats. It has been alpha-tested in the Phil Johnson Library of the AIDS Resource Center in Dallas, Texas, and refined through an iterative process over time.

INTENDED AUDIENCE

HIV/AIDS and HIV/AIDS-Related Terminology: A Means of Organizing the Body of Knowledge is designed for use by any organization or institution providing services related to HIV/ AIDS and requiring current information on this rapidly evolving field. Such organizations include but are not limited to community-based organizations, counseling centers, clinics, schools, family planning centers, AIDS service organizations, treatment centers, and libraries and information centers. The system can also be helpful to persons who maintain a private library or file of HIV/AIDS materials. In short, this structured vocabulary is intended for use by individuals in any arena concerned with the creation, collection, organization, management, or dissemination of HIV/AIDS-related information and materials.

STRUCTURE OF THE WORK

This work is divided into Instructions for Use, Domains and Headings, and Alphabetical Index. Within the Domains and Headings are ten broad subject areas under which specific terms are arranged hierarchically. Also included are Universal Subdivisions, designed to be applied as needed to headings to facilitate access to the information. It is hoped that this arrangement is sufficiently flexible to allow adaptation to individual needs and settings.

Indeed, since AIDS medicine changes daily, and the information associated with it is epidemic in growth, considerable latitude must be left in any arrangement to allow for its continued usefulness in light of the changes that will undoubtedly occur. Grouping and classification schemes may emerge from this structured vocabulary in response to individual settings and needs; furthermore, individuals using this tool are encouraged to add terms to the appropriate place in the hierarchy as the AIDS vernacular grows and changes.

HIV/AIDS and HIV/AIDS-Related Terminology: A Means of Organizing the Body of Knowledge is offered in the hope that the timely provision of accurate information will lighten the burden of all those affected by the epidemic and the terrible toll it exacts from patients, caregivers, families, friends, and society.

Instructions for Use

ARRANGEMENT OF THE WORK

The main body of this work consists of two key components: a structured vocabulary arranged hierarchically, and an alphabetical index that refers users to the appropriate term and its respective placement in the hierarchy. The hierarchical arrangement is divided into ten broad domains. Domains are subdivided further using headings and subheadings, thus producing a taxonomic classification system. This arrangement establishes the relationship of terms relative to one another. Contained in a universal subdivision subsection of the hierarchical arrangement are terms commonly associated with various issues concerning HIV/AIDS. Universal subdivisions may be added wherever appropriate to describe the subject of a work.

The alphabetical listing consists of all terms included in the hierarchical arrangement as well as variations of those terms. This section refers users to the appropriate term and its position within the hierarchy. The alphabetical listing includes cross references (SEE, SEE ALSO references) to facilitate access to information contained in the hierarchical structure.

DESCRIPTION OF TERMINOLOGY

Terminology included in this work reflects the most common form as evidenced in the HIV/AIDS literature. The following are examples of preferred forms:

- Preferred plural forms; e.g., Lentiviruses rather than Lentivirus;
- Preferred Anglicized term rather than Latin; e.g., Lentiviruses rather than Lentiviridae;
- Preferred normal word order rather than inverted word order; e.g., cell-mediated immunity rather than Immunity, cellular*. (MeSH terms are often inverted and are identified with an asterisk.)

Proper names, names of institutions and organizations, drug names, and names of special events generally have not been included in this work. This is an intentional omission in an effort to simplify use of this tool due to the constant flux within this vocabulary. These names should be included by users as necessary in the appropriate place in the hierarchical arrangement. The following are examples of possible name additions:

- Add Hemlock Society as a specific organization to Agencies and Organizations under Dying, Death, Bereavement in the Psychosocial and Religious Issues, Case Management domain;
- Add Americans with Disabilities Act as a specific law to Laws under Legislation and Jurisprudence in the Legal, Ethical, Economic, Political Aspects domain;
- Add NAMES Project as a specific organization under AIDS Service Organizations in the Organizations, Funding Opportunities, and Health Policy domain.

RULES FOR DESCRIPTION

Choose the most specific term or terms possible when describing a work. Multiple subject headings may be used to facilitate access to the information. Choose as many as needed to describe materials, so that users will be directed to things they need. As a general rule, choose no more than five main terms. In combining subject headings and universal subdivisions, the following punctuation is suggested:

- Separate subject headings using dashes (–);
- Separate subject headings and universal subdivisions with a forward slash (/).

It may be necessary to alter suggested punctuation when using certain software packages for information management.

Subject headings may be combined with one another to represent topics adequately. A secondary concept may be added to a main subject heading using dashes (–). For example:

- Acquired Immunodeficiency Syndrome–Epidemiology
- Prostitution–Education and Prevention
- Mycobacterium Avium Complex–Complications–Drug Therapy
- Thalidomide–Administration and Dosage–Adverse Effects

RULES FOR USE OF UNIVERSAL SUBDIVISIONS

After selecting subject headings, universal subdivisions may be applied to describe the work more fully. Universal subdivisions should be attached to subject headings using a forward slash (/). For example:

- Behavioral Factors in Transmission/Bisexual
- Seroprevalence/Uganda
- Cryptosporidiosis/Signs and Symptoms
- HIV-1–Transmission/Adolescent.

Apply the most specific geographic subdivision that describes the work and distinguishes the geographic location. For major cities of the world, use the name of the city without the name of the country. For example, use Paris for Paris, France. However, distinguish Paris, Kentucky from Paris, France by including the name of the state.

- Paris
- Kentucky–Paris

CONCLUSION

This work is presented as a tool to be modified, as necessary, based on individual and institutional needs. Terms should be added as required. White space is included for notations in the margins of the work and additional pages are available following the Alphabetical Index for more extensive user notes.

Index of Domains and Main Headings

Generalities

Basic science
Basic medical science
HIV disease
Testing
Information resources
Consumer health
Reports, documents
Research*

Epidemiology and Transmission

Definition(s) (for HIV disease and AIDS)
Strains of HIV
Epidemiology
United States Statistics and Demographics
International Statistics and Demographics
Transmission*
Behavioral Factors in Transmission

Education and Prevention

Prevention
Outreach
Continuing Education
Continuing Education for Professions Other than Medical
Education during Training

Education for Other Adult Groups
Strategies, Curricula, Campaigns
Safe, Safer Sex
Safer Injection Drug Use
~Other Risk Behaviors
Infection Control*

Clinical Manifestations of HIV: Complications, Malignancies and Infections Associated with AIDS

Opportunistic Infections*
Bacterial Infections*
Cancers
Complications and Conditions
Fungal Infections
Protozoan Infections*
Viral Infections

Treatments and Therapies: Medical Management of HIV Disease

Vaccine Development
Drug Development
Clinical Trials*
Clinical Trial Protocols
Medical Management of HIV Disease
Dental Aspects
Nutrition*
Diet*
Alternative Medicine*

Psychosocial and Religious Issues, Case Management

Case Management
Psychology*
Services to HIV+ Individuals and PLWAs

Dying, Death, Bereavement
Family Aspects
Psychosocial Aspects
Religious and Spiritual Aspects

Legal, Ethical, Economic, Political Aspects

Legislation and Jurisprudence*
Legal Aspects
Ethical Aspects
Economic Aspects
Political Aspects
Insurance
Prejudice*
Sexual Harassment*
Workplace* (Other than Infection Control*)
Military Aspects

Organizations, Funding Opportunities, and Health Policy

Hotlines
Health Care Organizations
AIDS Service Organizations
~Other Private Organizations
United States Government
State Governments
Local Governments
International Agencies
Events
Contributions and Funding

Fine Arts

Music*
Dance
Performance Art

Posters
Photography*
Drawing
Painting
Sculpture*
Film
Television*

Belles Lettres and Nonfiction

Literature
Quotations
Fiction
Drama
Humor
Poetry*
Essays
Anthologies
Nonfiction
Juvenile Literature

Domains and Headings

SN: Scope Notes
*Indicates Medical Subject Heading (MeSH)
>Indicates near-equivalent Medical Subject Heading (MeSH)
~Indicates grouping term only, not to be used for indexing or cataloging

GENERALITIES

SN: This domain covers basic information about HIV/AIDS and very general works that cannot be more specifically indexed.

Basic science

Anatomy*
Biochemistry*
Biology*
Chemistry*
Endocrinology*
Genetics*
Hematology*
Histology*
Immunology*
  Cell-mediated immunity
Microbiology*
  Bacteriology*
  Mycology*
  Virology*
    Arenaviruses
    Filoviruses
      Ebola>

                Marburg
             Retroviruses>
               Lentiviruses>
                 HIV-1*
                   Structure of HIV-1 virion
                     Proteins*
                     Glycoproteins*
                     Lipids*
                     Reverse transcriptase*
                       Deoxyribonucleic acid
                       Ribonucleic acid
                 HIV-2*
                 SIV*
         Molecular biology*
         Pathology*
         Pharmacology*
         Physiology*

Basic medical science

SN: Include here works describing the place of any of these medical specialties in HIV disease and the spectrum of care.

   Cardiology*
   Dentistry*
   Dermatology*
   Endocrinology*
   Family practice*
   Gastroenterology*
   General internal medicine
   Gynecology*
   Hematology*
   Neonatology*
   Nephrology*
   Neurology*
   Neurosurgery*

Obstetrics*
Oncology
Ophthalmology*
Otolaryngology*
Orthopedics*
Pediatrics*
Podiatry*
Proctology
Psychiatry*
Pulmonology*
Radiology*
Surgery*
Urology*

HIV disease

Etiology*
   Theories
Infection*
   Pathogenesis

SN: Include here cellular responses to HIV infection.

Antibodies*
Antigens*
Proteins*
   Tumor necrosis factor*
Replication cycle
   Binding sites*
      CD4 receptors
      Macrophages*
         Monocytes*
      Dendrites*
   Reverse transcription
   Virus integration*
      Provirus>

       Genetic expression
         Enzymatic proteins
           Gag>
           Pol>
           Env>
         Regulatory gene products
           Tat>
           Rev>
           Nef>
         Assembly
         Budding
           Polyproteins
           Viral protease
         Maturation
     Seroconversion
       Seroreversion
       Window period
   HIV disease progression
     Host factors in HIV disease progression
     Categories of HIV disease progression
       Long term survivors
       Non-progressors
       Rapid progressors
       Cleared
     Cofactors in HIV disease progression
       Age as cofactor
       Complications, disease processes as cofactors

SN: Include here information on disease processes only as they relate to HIV disease progression. For information concerning complications or disease processes secondary to HIV infection, SEE specific complication, malignancy, or infection associated with AIDS.

      Bacterial infections as cofactors
      Cancers as cofactors
      Complications as cofactors
      Fungal infections as cofactors
      Protozoan infections as cofactors
      Virus diseases as cofactors
   Environmental cofactors

SN: Include here information discussing the possibility of environmental phenomena such as sunlight's contributing to the progression of HIV disease.

   Individual response as cofactor

SN: Include here information concerning the impact of an infected individual's general constitution as a cofactor in HIV disease progression.

   Psychosocial cofactors

SN: Include here information discussing the possibility of psychosocial events such as stress associated with any type of loss contributing to the progression of HIV disease.

 HIV disease progression predictors
  Diversity threshold
  Surrogate markers as predictors
   Laboratory tests as predictors
    Anergy as predictor
    Beta microglobulin as predictor
    CD4-CD8 ratio as predictor
    Neopteria as predictor
    Quantitative, qualitative viral analysis as predictor
   Viral load as predictor
  Symptomatic indicators as predictors
   Dermatological indicators as predictors
   Neurological indicators as predictors
    Cognitive changes as predictors
    Memory loss as predictor

Metabolic indicators as predictors
 Fatigue as predictor
 Fever as predictor
 Muscular atrophy as predictor
 Night sweats as predictor
 Weight loss as predictor

Testing

Issues in testing
 Anonymous testing
 Confidentiality*
 Counseling in testing
  Pre-test
  Seronegative post-test
  Seropositive post-test
  Partners
  Family members
  Models
 Indications for seeking, recommending testing
 Informed consent in testing
 Mandatory testing
  Premarital testing
  Testing after delivery
  Testing during pregnancy
 Partner notification
  Contact tracing*
 Pregnancy testing

SN: Include here works concerning testing for pregnancy, not testing for HIV seropositivity.

 Surveillance reporting
 Voluntary testing
Types of test results
 Positive test

Negative test
False positive test
False negative test
Indeterminate test

HIV antibody testing
Enzyme-linked immunosorbent assay
Rapid EIA test
Combination ELISA test
Western blot assay
HIV antigen assay
Viral culture
Polymerase chain reaction*
DNA sequencing
RNA testing
Alternative tests
Home test kits
Saliva tests
Urine tests

Information resources

SN: Include here where appropriate works concerning the information resources (e.g., product documentation, product/system reviews, etc.).

~Print sources
Almanacs*
Atlases*

SN: Include here medical as well as geographic atlases.

Bibliographies
Bibliometrics*
Biobibliography*
Dictionaries*
Directories*

Encyclopedias*
Glossaries
Handbooks*
Indexes*
Medical reference books
Medical textbooks
Resource guides
Thesauri
Theses

SN: Include here both master's theses and doctoral dissertations.

Audio-Visual resources
    Audio information resources
        Audiocassette tapes
        Audio CD-ROM

SN: Include here compact disks containing audio only.

Visual resources
    Filmstrips*
    Medical models
    Microscope slides
    Motion pictures
    Overhead transparencies
    Photographic slides
    Videotape recordings*
Electronic and telecommunication sources, computer technology
    Internet

SN: Include here works on gopher, Mosaic, Lynx, World Wide Web (WWW), WAIS, and other evolving tools and interfaces as well as general works about the Internet.

        Computer bulletin boards
        Lists and discussion lists
        Electronic serials
        Other

Hotlines*
Computer applications
  Software*
  CD-ROM computer applications

SN: Include here all CD-ROMS that are not audio and not multi-media.

  Multimedia
    CD-ROM multimedia resources

SN: Include here all compact/CD-ROM products other than audio or strictly audio-visual CD-ROMS.

    Laserdisks
    Other

  Medical informatics*

SN: Include here works concerning the use of computer technology to enhance the delivery of health care.

    Computer-based patient record
    Decision support systems
      Therapy
      Management
      Wellness
    Computer simulations>

Computer systems*
  Computer communication networks*
    Local area networks*
  Computer peripherals*
  Microcomputers*
  Minicomputers*
  Mainframe computers

Electronic databases
  Security of electronic databases

Documentation*
  Abstracting and indexing*
  Cataloging*
  Filing*
  Subject headings*

PLWA alternative treatment information network

Library and information networks

Library and information services
  Library administration*
  Library associations*
  Library automation*
  Information centers*
  Library collection development*
  Library services*
    Public library services

SN: Include here works concerned with any facet of traditional and nontraditional public services in any library setting.

    Technical library services

SN: Include here works concerned with any facet of traditional and nontraditional technical services in any library setting.

    Information access
    Information management
    Information dissemination

  Catalogs*

Consumer Health

SN: Include here popular or lay works, especially those devoted to patient education.

Reports, documents

Conference proceedings

SN: Include here not only the proceedings and published abstracts themselves but also notes.

Congresses*

Letters

Obituaries

Public opinion*

Questionnaires*
Reports
Surveys

Resolutions

Research*

SN: Included here are terms applied to various types of biomedical research. Use in combination with the actual topic of the research.

Animal*

SN: Apply if research was conducted only on animal subjects. If not included, assume that the subjects of the research were human.

Mathematical models
Statistical models>
Forecasting*

~Publication types
Case studies*

    Controlled clinical trials*
      Meta-analysis*
      Multicenter AIDS cohort studies
      Randomized controlled trials*
        Double-blind>
      Reviews
      Twin studies*

  ~Other publication types

SN: Include here journal articles, government publications, or other documents considered relevant to HIV disease and that match the criteria for these categories.

    Classical articles
SN: Seminal document on a topic.

    Historical articles

SN: Documents whose subjects are past events. Distinguish from Review, which is a summation of research into a given area up to a particular point in time.

    Practice guidelines*

SN: Often emerging from Concensus Development Conferences, these documents give practical and specific direction for all areas of health care, but especially for treatment. Usually these will be government documents.

    Predictive value of tests*

EPIDEMIOLOGY AND TRANSMISSION

Definition(s) (for HIV infection and AIDS)

    Classification of HIV disease
    Definition of AIDS
    Staging of HIV disease

Strains of HIV

HIV-1*
HIV-2*
HTLV I/II

Epidemiology*

Incidence*
Index case
Prevalence*
Future projections

United States Statistics and Demographics

SN: Use universal subdivisions as appropriate.

Seroprevalence in United States
PLWAs in United States
Morbidity in United States
Mortality in United States
Future projections in United States

International Statistics and Demographics

SN: Use universal subdivisions as appropriate.

Seroprevalence in world
PLWAs in world '
Morbidity in world
Mortality in world
Future projections in world

Transmission*

SN: Include here only works concerning the transmission of HIV. For transmission of infections secondary to HIV, SEE specific disease, complication, or opportunistic infection.

Body fluids and by-products

SN: Use for general articles about transmission via one or more of these means.

Blood*
Breast milk
Feces*
Mucosal secretions
Perspiration
Pre-ejaculatory secretions
Saliva*
Semen*
Tears*
Urine*

Injection drug use
Shooting galleries

Occupational exposure*
Embalming*
Dentistry*
Human bites>
Laboratories*
Needlestick injuries*
Surgery*
Other

Perinatal exposure
Exposure in utero
Exposure during delivery
Caesarean section
Vaginal delivery

Behavioral Factors in Transmission

Substance abuse*
Alcohol and other non-injection drug use

Injection drug use
    Booting
    Needle sharing*

Sexual behaviors

SN: For specific sexual behaviors and their assumed degrees of risk, SEE Safe, Safer Sex.

EDUCATION AND PREVENTION

Prevention

SN: Include here works of a general nature concerning prevention strategies, educational approaches, or related topics.

Outreach

SN: Include here works concerning outreach in any form, including contact with researchers, individuals in affected communities, etc.

Continuing Education

SN: Include here works concerning education for degreed or certified practitioners.

Continuing education for medical professions
    Continuing education for medical specialties
    Continuing education for nursing
    Continuing education for dentistry
    Continuing education for pharmacy

Continuing education for allied health professions
    Audiology*
    Continuing education for nutrition
    Dental technology
    Dietetics*

Emergency medical technicians*
Medical records services
Medical technology
Mental health personnel
   Continuing education for psychology
   Continuing education for social work
Occupational therapy*
Physical therapy*
Physician assistants*
Public health*
Radiology technology
Rehabilitation therapy
Respiratory therapy*
Speech and language pathology
Other

Continuing education for professions other than medical

Anthropology*
Clergy*
Mortuary science
Social work*
Other

Education
   Administrators
   Board members
   Support staff
   Teachers
Information professionals

~Education during training

SN: Include here works concerning education for students pre-
paring to enter a professional medical or allied health field.

Medical school education>

Nursing school education>

Dental school education>

Pharmacy school education>

Allied health education

Other

~Education for other adult groups

Lay public

Workplace education

Strategies, curricula, campaigns

SN: Include here all levels of curricula, including those intended for continuing education for professionals.

Human sexuality education
   Lesson plans

Safe, safer sex education

SN: Include here works concerning both the education of individuals at risk for infection with HIV and those who are infected.

Relapse

Community health initiatives

Substance abuse*
   Alcohol and other non-injection drug use
   Injection drug use
   Needle exchange programs

Family planning*
   Contraceptive devices*
   Pregnancy*

Schools*
  Preschools
  Elementary schools
    Primary schools
    Intermediate schools
  Middle schools
  Secondary schools
  Postsecondary schools

Teaching methods
  Peer education
  Other

Safe, safer sex

Sex behaviors>

Low risk sex behaviors

SN: Low risk activities performed with partners' touching one another and with the use of a prophylactic such as a condom.

    Abstinence
    Closed mouth kissing
    Digital intercourse
      Anal digital intercourse
      Vaginal digital intercourse
    Eroticism

SN: Refers to the use of erotic or pornographic material for sexual arousal without engaging in higher risk activities.

    Eroticism with partner
    Frottage

    Manual intercourse
      Anal manual intercourse
      Vaginal manual intercourse

Masturbation*
 Individual masturbation
 Mutual masturbation

Monogamy

SN: Include here works concerning a long-term relationship between two mutually faithful individuals.

Storytelling

SN: Include here works concerning partners' verbal sharing of erotic fantasies or desires.

Touch*

SN: Include here non-sexual massage, hugging, etc.

Protected sexual practices
 Protected oral-genital sex
 Protected anilingus
 Protected cunnilingus
 Protected fellatio

Protected sexual intercourse

SN: Include here works concerning protected vaginal or anal intercourse with a latex or polyurethane condom.

Protected insertive anal intercourse
 Protected receptive anal intercourse
 Protected vaginal intercourse

High risk sex behaviors
 Water sports

SN: Sometimes called "golden shower." Include here works concerning contact with partner's urine.

Bathhouses

SN: Include here works concerning high risk behaviors frequently practiced in these establishments.

Unprotected sexual practices
Unprotected oral-genital sex
Unprotected anilingus
Unprotected cunnilingus
Unprotected fellatio

Unprotected sexual intercourse
Unprotected insertive anal intercourse
Unprotected receptive anal intercourse
Unprotected vaginal intercourse

Resources for safe, safer sex
Communication*
Negotiation

Products for safe, safer sex
Spermicides
Lubricants
Water-based lubricants
Oil-based lubricants
Other lubricants

Devices for safe, safer sex
Condoms*
Latex condoms
Female latex condoms
Male latex condoms
Polyurethane condoms
Female polyurethane condoms
Male polyurethane condoms

Condom distribution programs
Condom use
Condom efficacy

Dental dams

Sex toys and paraphernalia

Safer injection drug use

Resources for safer injection drug use
    Needle exchange programs
    Needle cleaning
      Bleach kits

~Other risk behaviors

Body modification
    Piercing
    Tattooing*
    Other

Circumcision*

SN: Include here works concerning circumcision, male or female, after infancy.

*Infection Control**

Universal precautions*
    Clinics
    Health clubs
    Hospitals*
    Households
    Nursing homes*
    Schools*
    Other environments

Fluid, organ, tissue banks
    Blood and blood product banks>
    Milk banks
    Organ banks
    Sperm banks*
      Ejaculation*
    Tissue banks*

CLINICAL MANIFESTATIONS OF HIV: COMPLICATIONS, MALIGNANCIES, AND INFECTIONS ASSOCIATED WITH AIDS

Opportunistic Infections*

SN: Include here general works and review articles which encompass a spectrum of infections.

Bacterial Infections*

Bacterial infections, general works

Anthrax*
Bacillary angiomatosis
Bacillary dysentery>
Bacterial pneumonia>
Cat scratch disease>
Chlamydia infections*
Cholera*
Gonorrhea*
Leprosy*
Listeria infections*

Mycobacterium avium complex*

SN: For infections, use Mycobacterium avium-intracellulare infection*.

Mycobacterium avium-intracellulare infection*
  Mycobacterium kansasii
  Mycobacterium tuberculosis*

Ornithosis*
Salmonella infections*
  Typhoid*
Septic shock>

Syphilis*
   Cardiovascular syphilis>
   Neurosyphilis*
Tuberculosis*
   Multidrug-resistant tuberculosis
Typhus

Cancers

Cancers, general works

Basal cell carcinoma>
Breast neoplasms*
Cervix neoplasms*
Kaposi's sarcoma>
Leukemia*
Lymphoma*
   AIDS-related lymphoma>
   Burkitt's lymphoma*
   Hodgkin's disease*
   Non-Hodgkin's lymphoma>
   Sezary syndrome*
Squamous cell carcinoma>
Testicular neoplasms*

Complications and Conditions

Complications, general works

Abscess*
Acquired immunodeficiency syndrome*
   AIDS prodrome
Addison's disease*
Adenopathy
   Lymphadenopathy

AIDS dementia complex*

AIDS-related complex*

SN: For historical use only. Otherwise, use Lymphadenopathy.

Alcoholism*
Allergy
Alopecia*
Anorectal disease
Anorexia*
Anoxia*
Atrophy*
  Testicular atrophy

Blood-brain barrier*
Cavitary lesion
Cerebrovascular disorders*
Cheilitis*
Chorioretinitis*

Coronary disease*
  Congestive cardiomyopathy
  Myocardial infarction*
  Endocarditis*
  Myocarditis*
  Pericarditis*

Cotton-wool spots

Decubitus ulcer*

Dermatologic disorders
  Acute HIV exanthem
  Atopic diathesis

  Dermatitis*
    Atopic dermatitis
    Drug eruptions*
    Seborrheic dermatitis

Ecthyma*
Ichthyosis*
Impetigo*
Intertrigo*
Mange
Molluscum contagiosum*
Psoriasis*
Scabies*
   Norwegian scabies
Stevens-Johnson syndrome*
Yellow nail syndrome

Disease susceptibility*
Eating disorders*
Edema*
Epistaxis*
Erythema multiforme*
Fever*
   Fever of unknown origin*
Furunculosis*

Gastrointestinal disorders
   Achlorhydria*
   AIDS enteropathy
   Colitis*
   Diarrhea*
   Enteritis*
   Esophagitis*
   Helminthiasis*
   Inflammatory bowel diseases*
   Proctitis*
      Proctocolitis*
   Reye's syndrome*
   Strongyloidiasis*

Gynecologic disorders
  Cervix dysplasia*
  Fibrocystic breasts>
  Mastitis*
  Menstruation*
    Amenorrhea*
    Dysmenorrhea*
  Pelvic inflammatory disease*
  Pregnancy complications*
  Vaginitis*

Headache*

Hematologic disorders
  Anemia*
    Sickle cell trait*
  Bacteremia*
  Hemophilia*
    Factor VIII*
  Neutropenia*
  Thrombocytopenia*
  von Willebrand's disease*

Hepatomegaly*
Hypercapnia*
Hyperplasia*
Hypertension*
Hyperthermia*
Hypertrophy*
Hypoglycemia*
Hypogonadism*
Hyponatremia*
Hypotension*
Hypothermia*
Hypovolemia
Idiopathic CD4+ T lymphocytopenia

Idiopathic thrombocytopenic purpura>
Immune thrombocytopenic purpura>
Impotence*
Incontinence
Ischemia*
Jaundice*
Leukopenia*
Light sensitivity

SN: Include here works referring to sensitivity to brightness of any kind of light, not just sunlight. SEE Photosensitivity disorders* for skin problems associated with light.

Malnutrition

Meningitis*

SN: Some diseases (e.g., meningitis), take different forms and have different causative agents; they have their own heading. Those forms specific to AIDS patients are found under the broad heading of Fungal Infections.

Mental disorders*
    Anxiety*
    Denial*
    Depression*
    Obsessive-compulsive disorder*
    Post traumatic stress disorder>
    Sleep disorders*

Metabolic disorders
    Amyloidosis*
    Diabetes insipidus*
    Diabetes mellitus*
    Hyperglycemia*
    Malabsorption syndromes*
      Celiac disease*
      Whipple's disease

Metabolic acidosis
Water-electrolyte imbalance*
   Hyperkalemia*
   Hypokalemia*

Myositis*
Necrosis*

Neurologic disorders
   Apoplexy
   Cranial nerve palsy
   Creutzfeld-Jakob syndrome*
   Delirium*
   Distal symmetric polyneuropathy
   Facial nerve diseases*
   Facial paralysis*
   HIV encephalopathy
     Metabolic encephalopathy
   Kuru*
   Neuropathy
   Seizures*
   Transient ischemic attack

Nocardia infections*

SN: Infections are caused by a genus transitional between bacteria and fungi.

Nutrition disorders*
   Vitamin deficiencies

Ophthalmologic disorders
   Chorioretinitis*
   Cotton-wool spots

Oral disorders
   Aphthous stomatitis
   Aphthous ulcer

Dysphagia
Leukoplakia*
Hairy leukoplakia>

SN: Specific form of oral leukoplakia commonly seen in HIV-infected individuals. Lesions most often occur on the lateral margins of the tongue.

Oral leukoplakia>

SN: Generally benign lesion that may occur on any mucous membrane but is commonly seen in the mouths of HIV-infected individuals. It may represent a pre-cancerous condition. Some references associate it with the Epstein-Barr virus.

Salivary gland diseases*

Periodontal diseases*

SN: For inflammations, use Periodontitis*.

Periodontitis*

Osteomyelitis*

Otorhinolaryngologic disorders
Otitis media*
Mastoiditis*
Rhinitis*
Sinusitis*

Pain*
Arthralgia*

Pancreatitis*
Parotitis*
Peritonitis*

Photosensitivity disorders*

SN: Include here works concerning skin problems associated with light.

Porphyria*

Pneumonia*
  Lymphocytic interstitial pneumonia

Respiration disorders*
  Adult respiratory distress syndrome>
  Apnea*
  Asthma*
  Bronchitis*
  Dyspnea*
  Idiopathic inflammatory pulmonary disease
  Pulmonary alveolar proteinosis*

Respiratory distress syndrome*

SN: Use only for infants.

Reiter's disease*
Schistosomiasis*

Sexually transmitted diseases*

SN: Include here works whose general focus is several or all STDs.

Sleep disorders*
  Sleep apnea>
  Insomnia*

Spinal cord disorders
  Myelitis*
  Spinal muscular atrophy>
  Myelopathy
    Vacuolar myelopathy

Splenomegaly*
Syncope*

Ulcer*

SN: Include here works having to do with ulcers anywhere on or in the body, with the exception of Decutibus ulcer*.

Uremia*
Urethritis*
Wasting syndrome

Fungal Infections

Fungal infections, general works

Aspergillosis*
Candidiasis*
   Atrophic candidiasis
   Chronic mucocutaneous candidiasis>
   Cutaneous candidiasis>
   Hyperplastic candidiasis
   Oral candidiasis>
   Vulvovaginal candidiasis>

Coccidioidomycosis*
   Valley fever
Cryptococcal meningitis>
Cryptococcosis*
Histoplasmosis*
Pneumocystis carinii pneumonia>
Sporotrichosis*
Tinea*
   Tinea pedis*

*Protozoan Infections**

Protozoan infections, general works

Amebiasis*
Coccidiosis*
Cryptosporidiosis*
Elephantiasis*
Giardiasis*
Microsporidiosis

Toxoplasmosis*
Trichomonas infections*

Viral Infections

Viral infections, general works

Adenovirus infections>
African swine fever*
Aphthovirus*
Arenavirus infections>
Chronic fatigue syndrome>
Encephalitis*

Hantavirus*

SN: Include here works on both hantavirus and epidemic hemorrhagic fever.

Hepatitis*

SN: Include here general works on hepatitis, including works specifically about one or all types of hepatitis, A-E, except for hepatitis B.

Hepatitis B*

Herpesvirus

Cytomegalovirus infections*

SN: Include here works on cytomegalovirus infections as well as cytomegalic inclusion disease.

Cytomegalovirus retinitis*

Polyradiculopathy
   Lumbosacral polyradiculopathy

Epstein-Barr virus
   Infectious mononucleosis*

Herpes simplex*
   Genital herpes simplex
   Oral herpes simplex

Herpes zoster*
Varicella zoster

Human papilloma virus>
Influenza*
Lassa fever*
Progressive multifocal leukoencephalopathy>

TREATMENTS AND THERAPIES: MEDICAL MANAGEMENT OF HIV INFECTION

Vaccine Development

Agent
Adjuvant
AIDS Vaccine Evaluation Group

Drug Development

SN: Include here works concerning the research and development phase of pharmaceuticals used in the prevention and management of HIV infection.

Clinical Trials*

Drug approval*
    Investigational New Drug Application*
    AIDS Clinical Trials Group
    Clinical trials Phase I*
    Clinical trials Phase II*
    Clinical trials Phase III*
    Clinical trials Phase IV*

Alternative access
    Compassionate use

Expanded access
Open label protocol
Parallel track initiative

Clinical Trial Protocols

SN: Include here works concerning the purpose, structure, and administration of clinical trials of drugs, including participant inclusion/exclusion criteria.

Medical Management of HIV Disease

Diagnosis*
   Differential diagnosis*
   Presumptive diagnosis

Prognosis*
Medical history taking*
Early intervention
   Baseline studies

Triage*
   Telephone triage

Therapy*

   Dialysis*
      Hemodialysis*
      Peritoneal dialysis*
         Chronic ambulatory peritoneal dialysis

   Diet therapy*

   Drug therapy*

SN: Names of specific drugs are not included in this hierarchy. They should be added as needed.

Adverse effects*

Administration and dosage*

SN: Include here works concerning the way drugs are administered to patients and dosage levels.

Chemotherapy

Combination therapy
   Double therapy
   Multiple therapy
   Multiple therapy with protease inhibitor

Monotherapy

Viral resistance
Hormone therapy
Vitamin therapy

Genetic Techniques
   Gene amplification*
   Gene therapy*
      Antiviral gene therapy
      CD4-based gene therapy
      Cellular immunotherapy
   Genetic engineering*
      Antisense elements (genetics)*

Intensive care*

SN: Limit to any aspect of receiving specialized medical care in any intensive care unit of a hospital. Includes cardiac intensive care.

Pain management
   Analgesics*
Prevention of Infection
   Bacterial infection prevention
   Cancer prevention
   Complications prevention

    Fungal infection prevention
    Protozoan infection prevention
    Virus disease prevention

Primary care

Total parenteral nutrition>

Transplants

Treatment Protocols

SN: Include here specific regimens of therapy. May include drug therapy, diet therapy, physical therapy, psychotherapy, and other relevant holistic approaches tied to a protocol.

Vaccinations and immunizations
    BCG vaccine*
    Influenza vaccine*
    Hepatitis vaccine*
    Measles vaccine*
    Mumps vaccine*
    Pneumonia vaccine
    Rubella vaccine*
    Vaccination of HIV-infected children

Tests and Procedures

Laboratory tests

    Clinical chemistry
        Blood sugar test
        Cholesterol and lipids test
        Electrolytes*
        Hormone tests
        Kidney function tests*
        Liver function tests*
        Thyroid function tests*
        Urinalysis*
        Vitamin B-12 tests

Hematologic tests*
  Complete blood cell count
    Erythrocyte count*
      Reticulyte count*
    Leukocyte count*
      Lymphocytic count*
        CD4 lymphocyte count*
          T lymphocyte differential
          CD4 percentage
          CD4-CD8 ratio*
      Platelet count*

  Blood coagulation tests*
  Bone marrow examination*
  Erythrocyte aggregation*
  Erythrocyte indices*
  Erythrocyte sedimentation rate
  Hematocrit*
  Osmotic fragility*
  Schilling test*

  Immunologic tests*
    Coombs' test*
    Immunofluorescence assay
    Radioimmunoassay*
      Radioimmunoprecipitation assay*

Skin tests
  Tuberculin test*

Syphilis serodiagnosis*
  Venereal disease research laboratory test
  Other

Urine tests
  Urinalysis*
  Creatinine*

Creatinine clearance
Other

Culture and sensitivity
    Blood culture and sensitivity
    Bone marrow culture and sensitivity
    Bronchial culture and sensitivity
    Cerebrospinal fluid culture and sensitivity
    Gastric culture and sensitivity
    Genital culture and sensitivity
    Nasopharyngeal culture and sensitivity
    Sinus culture and sensitivity
    Sputum culture and sensitivity
    Stool culture and sensitivity
    Throat culture and sensitivity
    Urine culture and sensitivity

Procedures
    Abortion*
    Amniocentesis*
    Bioelectrical impedance analysis
    Biopsy*
    Bone marrow aspiration
    Bronchoalveolar lavage
    Bronchoscopy*
    Colposcopy*
    Diagnostic imaging*
        Computerized axial tomographic scan>
        Echocardiography*
        Mammography*
        Magnetic resonance imaging*
        Positron emission tomography>
        Radiographic assessment
        Ultrasonography*

Enema*
First aid*
Laser therapy
Mechanical ventilation>
Respiration, artificial*
Sigmoidoscopy*

Genital self-examination

Cytodiagnosis*
  Pap smear
  Spinal puncture*
  Vaginal smears*

Radiation therapy

Nursing Perspective
Nursing assessment*
  Physical examination*
Nursing diagnosis*
Nursing intervention
  Nursing protocols
Nursing evaluation

Dental aspects

SN: Include here works concerning the dental care of HIV-infected individuals.

Nutrition*

SN: Include here nutritional values and benefits of categories of foods or specific foods.

Diet*

SN: Include here what and when one eats, quantities, recipes, and menus.

Macrobiotic diet>
Vegetarian diet
Beverages*
    Drinking water
Menus
Recipes

Exercise*

Alternative Medicine*

SN: Alternative approaches to treatment of HIV infection evolve continuously. Broad categories are outlined in this scheme, with some alternative therapies named. As new therapies are made available, add them under the headings as needed.

Immune system enhancement, general well-being

SN: Include here only the most general works.

Nutritional, Herbal Therapies
    Nutritional supplements
        Vitamin therapy

SN: Add names of vitamins as needed, e.g., Vitamin C, Vitamin B-12.

        Mineral therapy

SN: Add names of minerals as needed, e.g., Selenium.

        Other

Medicinal plants>
    Alfalfa*
    Aloe*
    Astragalus
    Cannabis*
    Echinacea
    Eucalyptus*

    Garlic*
    Ginseng*
    GLQ-223
    Licorice
    Mistletoe
    Mushrooms
      Kambucha tea mushroom
    Spirulina
    Other

Mind, Body, Spirit Connection
  Holistic health*
    Hypnotherapy
    Psychoneuroimmunology*

  Sensory, creative therapies
    Aroma therapy
    Art therapy*
    Color therapy*
    Drama therapy
    Music therapy*
    Play therapy*
    Therapeutic touch*

  Movement therapies
    Dance therapy*
    Tai chi
    Yoga*

  Coping therapies
    Bibliotherapy*
      Poetry therapy
    Biofeedback>
    Guided imagery
    Humor therapy
    Stress reduction
    Visualization

Philosophical, spiritual therapies
  Meditation
  Theosophy
    Anthroposophy*

Traditional, Ethnomedical Approaches
  African traditional medicine
  Ayurvedic medicine>
  Homeopathy*
  Native American traditional medicine
  Naturopathy*
  Oriental traditional medicine>
    Acupressure*
    Acupuncture*

    Chinese traditional medicine>
      Yin-Yang*
  Shamanism

Manipulative, Energetic Therapies
  Chiropractic*
  Kinesiology

  Massage*
    Swedish massage
    Reiki massage
    Shiatzu massage
    Rolfing massage
    Other massage

  Osteopathic medicine*
  Reflexology

Pharmacological, Biological Therapies
  Pharmacological therapies
    Anabolic steroids*
    Antioxidants*

Oxidizers
Hydrogen peroxide*
Ozone*

Biological therapies
Induced hyperthermia>
Iridology

Bioelectromagnetic Therapies
Artificial lighting
Blue light treatment
Electromagnetic fields*
Electrostimulation, neuromagnetic stimulation devices
Magnetoresonance spectroscopy

PSYCHOSOCIAL AND RELIGIOUS ISSUES, CASE MANAGEMENT

Case Management

Psychology*

SN: For clinical treatment of specific psychological disorders, see under Medical Management. Include here models for treating various groups of individuals and general counseling/psychotherapy concerns.

Psychological models

Individual psychological treatment models
Counseling*
Hypnosis*
Psychoanalysis*

Group psychological treatment models
Support groups
Therapy groups

Professional issues
   Burnout>
   Countertransference
   Transference>

Self-help
   Addiction disorders
      Sexual addiction disorders
      Relationship addiction disorders
      Substance addiction disorders
      Other addiction disorders
   Addictive behavior>
   Psychological self-help
   Recovery

Services to HIV+ Individuals and PLWAs

Dating services
Household services
   Cleaning services
   Maintenance services
   Pet care services
   Plant care services
Child care services
Legal assistance services

SN: Include here information about services. For legal issues affecting individuals infected with HIV, use Legal Aspects.

Financial assistance services
Personal services
   Clothing exchanges
   Nutrition services
   Emergency food services
   Delivered meals
   Other services

Housing assistance services
Medical assistance services>
  Buyers' clubs
  Insurance services
  Medicaid*
  Medicare*
AIDS care services
  Assisted living services
    AIDS group homes
  Buddy programs
  Home health agencies>
  Hospice services>
  Home-based services
  Medical
    Doctor-patient relations>
      Patient autonomy
    Inpatient services
  Nursing home services>

Dying, Death, Bereavement

Death counseling
  Death with dignity
  Denial of death
  Near-death experiences
  Permission to die
  Right to die*

Psychological preparation for death
  Patient preparation for death
  Partner preparation for death
  Family preparation for death
  Community preparation for death

Death*
  Autopsy*

Codes
  Code blue
  No code blue
  Do not resuscitate
  Euthanasia*
  Suicide*
    Assisted suicide>

Funeral preparation
  Cremation
  Embalming*
  Interment
  Memorial service
  Religious service

Bereavement*
  Stages of bereavement
Agencies and organizations
  Funeral homes
  Hospices*
  Religious entities

Family Aspects

Disclosure issues
  Coming out
    Sexual orientation
  Diagnosis disclosure
  Drug use disclosure
  Alcohol use disclosure
  Injection drug use disclosure
  Other drug use disclosure
  Other disclosure issues

Parenting*
  Parents of gays, lesbians

Gay, lesbian parents
Dysfunctional families
Family Constellations

SN: Any traditional or nontraditional unit or grouping of individuals living in a mutually acknowledged, committed relationship.

Collectives
Same-sex families
Traditional families

Marriage*

Divorce*

Children's Issues
Adoption of children>
Custody of children>
Foster care of children>
Orphans
Parental rights (severing)

Psychosocial Aspects

Quality of life*
Attitude*
Attitude to death*
Attitude to health*
Health behavior*
Patient acceptance of health care*
Patient compliance*
Patient satisfaction*
Treatment refusal*
Psychological adaptation>
Self-concept*
Self-disclosure*
Self-identity
Knowledge, attitudes, beliefs, behavior>

Religious and Spiritual Aspects

Personal religious and spiritual issues

SN: Include here individual issues associated with religion or spirituality. Consider self in relation to self and others. Apply universal subdivisions as needed.

Institutional religious and spiritual issues

SN: Include here works concerning stance or response issued by established religious organizations at any level (e.g., resolutions, proclamations, official statements, reports emanating from committees or task forces, etc.).

International religious organizations
National religious organizations
Regional religious organizations
Local religious organizations

Cultural religious and spiritual issues

SN: Include here works concerning sociological aspects of religion or spirituality, to include the underlying values, assumptions, and religious beliefs that are expressed by what the society is doing in response to the HIV/AIDS epidemic.

Religious scriptures
Religious cults

LEGAL, ETHICAL, ECONOMIC, AND POLITICAL ASPECTS

Legislation and Jurisprudence*

Bills

SN: Text of a document in legislative process; commentary on the documents.

Laws

SN: Text of a document that has been signed into law by the appropriate governmental figure; commentary on the laws.

Court cases

SN: Text of specific court decisions from any jurisdiction; commentary on the decisions.

Legal Aspects

Criminal
  Child abuse*
    Physical child abuse
    Sexual child abuse>
  Domestic abuse>
  Fraud*
  Intentional transmission of HIV
  Rape*
  Sale or possession of controlled substance
  Hate crimes
  Partner abuse
  Vandalism
  Other

Civil
  Advance directives*
    Power of attorney
      Durable power of attorney
        Durable power of attorney for health care
    Living wills*
  Censorship
  Civil Rights*
  Copyright issues>
  Death certificates*
  Discrimination

Emigration*
Immigration*
  Deportation
Informed consent*
Liability>
Mandatory education
Quarantine*
  Internment, internment camps
Sodomy

Ethical Aspects

Patient advocacy*
Patient empowerment

Economic Aspects

Costs>
  Cost-benefit analysis*
  Cost containment
  Health care costs*
Benefits
  Cash advances
  Government*
  Other benefits
Estate planning
  Beneficiaries
  Trusts
Resource allocation

Political Aspects

SN: Include here documents primarily concerned with political aspects of the epidemic, whether the political unit is international, federal, state, or local.

Executive branch
Legislative branch
Judicial branch

Political parties
   Democratic Party
   Republican Party
   Independent political parties
Government policy
Institutional policy
   Hospital policy
   Pharmaceutical company policy
   Health maintenance organization policy
   Other policy
Health care reform*

*Insurance**

Cost sharing*
Managed care>
Viatical benefits
Other insurance

*Prejudice**

AIDSphobia
Employment prejudice
Health care prejudice
   Medical professionals
Homophobia
   Gaybashing
Housing*
Organizations and prejudice
   Anti-gay
   Pro-gay
Public facilities and prejudice

Sexual Harassment*

Workplace* (Other than Infection Control*)

Employee Assistance Programs

Military Aspects

ORGANIZATIONS, FUNDING OPPORTUNITIES, AND HEALTH POLICY

Hotlines*

Crisis intervention*

Health Care Organizations

Policies of health care organizations
Procedures of health care organizations
  Security in health care organizations
Programs of health care organizations
Statistics of health care organizations
Strategic planning in health care organizations

~Types of health care organizations
  Hospitals*
  Health maintenance organizations*
  Extended care organizations
  Other health care organizations

AIDS Service Organizations

Policies of AIDS service organizations
Procedures of AIDS service organizations
  Security in AIDS service organizations
Programs of AIDS service organizations
Statistics of AIDS service organizations
Strategic planning in AIDS service organizations

~Other Private Organizations (e.g., AmFAR, American Red Cross)

    Policies of private organizations
    Procedures of private organizations
      Security in private organizations
    Programs of private organizations
    Statistics of private organizations
    Strategic planning in private organizations

United States Government

SN: This breakdown is not meant to be all-inclusive. The government agencies, bureaus, and offices most concerned with issues of HIV/AIDS have been included. Additional government entities may be added as necessary.

Health and Human Services>
    Administration on Aging
    Office for Civil Rights
    Office of Consumer Affairs

    Administration for Children and Families
    Health Care Financing Administration>
      Medicaid Bureau
    Public Health Service>
      Agency for Health Care Policy and Research>
      Substance Abuse and Mental Health Service Administration>
      Centers for Disease Control and Prevention>
      Food and Drug Administration>
      Health Resources and Services Administration>
        AIDS Program Office
        Office of Rural Health Policy
        Office of Minority Health
        Office of Public Health Practice

Bureau of Primary Health Care
Maternal and Child Health Bureau
Indian Health Service>
National Institutes of Health>
Office of AIDS Research
Office of Disease Prevention
Office of Research on Minority Health
Office of Research on Women's Health
Office of Behavioral and Social Sciences Research
National Cancer Institute
National Eye Institute
National Heart, Lung, and Blood Institute
National Institute on Aging
National Institute on Alcohol Abuse and Alcoholism
National Institute of Allergy and Infectious Diseases
National Institute of Arthritis and Musculoskeletal and
    Skin Diseases
National Institute of Child Health and Human Development
National Institute on Deafness and Other Communication
    Disorders
National Institute of Dental Research
National Institute of Diabetes and Digestive and Kidney
    Diseases
National Institute on Drug Abuse
National Institute of Environmental Health Sciences
National Institute of Mental Health>
National Institute of Neurological Disorders and Stroke
National Institute of Nursing Research
National Library of Medicine>
Fogarty International Center
National Center for Human Genome Research
Division of Research Grants

Social Security Administration>

Department of the Treasury
   Internal Revenue Service

Department of Education

Department of Defense

Department of Justice

Department of Labor
   Occupational Safety and Health Administration>

Department of the Interior

Department of Veterans' Affairs>

Environmental Protection Agency>

State Governments>

SN: Add names of states and state agencies as appropriate.

Local Governments

SN: Add names of local entities as appropriate.

   Regional governments
   County governments
   City governments

International Agencies*

SN: Add names of international entities as appropriate.

United Nations*
   World Health Organization*
      Assistance through World Health Organization
      Policies of World Health Organization
      Programs of World Health Organization
         Global Programme on AIDS

Events

SN: Include in all categories names of celebrities associated with the event.

Award ceremonies
Exhibits*
Fund raising*
   Benefits for fund raising
   Capital campaigns
   Special campaigns for fund raising
   Special events for fund raising

Activism
   Boycotts
   Demonstrations
   Protests
   Rallies
   Other activist activities

Contributions and Funding

Grants and contracts
   Proposal ideas
   Proposals in process
   Funded proposals
   Proposals submitted but not funded

Funding references

SN: Include here reference works that point researchers toward sources of funds, whether government, corporate, or foundation. Include here also works on how to develop proposals.

Funding sources
   Government funding sources
      Federal funding sources
      Regional funding sources

State funding sources
County funding sources
City funding sources

Foundation funding sources
International foundations
National foundations
State foundations
City foundations

Corporate funding sources

Individual funding sources

FINE ARTS

SN: Include here accounts of performances dedicated to PLWAs or persons lost to AIDS; distinguish from Benefits, which are performances used for fund-raising. Include here also actual works concerned with HIV, AIDS, the gay community, or other communities heavily impacted by the epidemic.

Music*

Instrumental music
Vocal music

Dance

Performance Art

Posters

Photography*

Drawing

Painting>

Sculpture*

Film

Television*

BELLES LETTRES AND NONFICTION

Literature*

SN: Include here works of a general literary character that do not conform to specified literary types.

Quotations

History and criticism

Fiction
    Story collections

SN: Include here fictional short stories or fictional compilations of vignettes concerning any aspect of HIV/AIDS or impacted populations.

Drama*

Humor*
    Cartoons

Poetry*

Essays

Anthologies

Nonfiction

Biography*, Autobiography*
  Collective Biography

SN: Include here biographical collections of sketches, vignettes, or studies concerning persons prominent in the epidemic, impacted populations, or relevant areas written or edited by an independent person. Distinguish from Personal narratives, Journals, Diaries, Interviews, which includes interviews or personal writings composed by individuals affected by HIV/AIDS.

Personal narratives, Journals, Diaries, Interviews

Meditations

History of AIDS Epidemic

History of Gay Liberation Movement

Herstory

SN: Include here history of the women's movement.

Other History

Women's Studies
  Feminism

Men's Studies

Gay, Lesbian Studies

Sociology*
  Communities
    Rural communities
    Suburban communities
    Urban communities
  Correctional facilities
  Drug culture
  Families
  Gay culture

Mass media*
Prostitution*

Anthropology*

Erotica*

Travel*

Sexuality
  Gay sexuality
  Lesbian sexuality
  Sadomasochism
  Transsexuality>
  Bisexuality*
  Heterosexuality

Juvenile Literature

Coloring books
Comic books

Universal Subdivisions

Age ranges

Neonate	Birth to 1 month
Infant*	1 through 23 months
Preschool child>	2 through 5 years
Child*	6 through 12 years
Adolescent>	13 through 18 years
Adult*	18 through 49 years
Middle age*	50 through 69 years
Aged*	70 years and over

Sexual orientation

Bisexual>
Heterosexual
Homosexual>
   Gay
   Lesbian

Gender

Female*
Male*
Transgendered

Stages of infection

HIV+ asymptomatic
HIV+ symptomatic
AIDS>

Ethnic groups*

SN: Where necessary for clarification, couple ethnic designation with country or region of origin (e.g., Asian/Middle East/Lebanon).

Asians
Blacks*
Central American Indians>
Hispanics
Nomadic Peoples
  Gypsies*
North American Indians>
Multi-ethnic
Pacific Islanders
South American Indians>
Whites*

SN: Include here individuals of Northern African descent (e.g., Egyptians).

Geographic names

SN: Not all countries in all regions are named. If a country is not named, use the regional designation. Add regional designations and city names as needed.

Africa*
  Northern Africa*
    Algeria*
    Egypt*
    Libya*
    Morocco*
    Tunisia*
  Sub-Saharan Africa*
    Cameroon*
    Central African Republic*
    Chad*
    Zaire*

Eastern Africa*
  Burundi*
  Ethiopia*
  Kenya*
  Rwanda*
  Somalia*
  Sudan*
  Tanzania*
  Uganda*
Western Africa*
  Ivory Coast>
  Gambia*
  Ghana*
  Liberia*
  Nigeria*
  Senegal*
Southern Africa*
  Angola*
  Botswana*
  Malawi*
  Mozambique*
  South Africa*
  Swaziland*
  Zimbabwe*

Asia*
  Southeastern Asia*
    Borneo*
    Burma*
    Cambodia*
    Indonesia*
    Laos*
    Malaysia*
    Philippines*
    Singapore*

      Thailand*
      Vietnam*
    Western Asia*
      Afghanistan*
      Bangladesh*
      India*
      Middle East*
        Arabian Peninsula*

SN: Include here all countries of the peninsula except Saudi Arabia.

        Iran*
        Iraq*
        Israel*
        Jordan*
        Lebanon*
        Saudi Arabia*
        Syria*
        Turkey*
      Pakistan*
      Sri Lanka*
    Far East*
      China*
      Hong Kong*

SN: When Hong Kong reverts to China in 1997, make the area subordinate to China.

      Japan*
      Korea*
      Taiwan*

Australia*

Europe*
    Eastern Europe*
      Albania*

Balkan States*
Baltic States*
Bulgaria*
Czech Republic*
Hungary*
Poland*
Romania*
Slovakia*
Ukraine*
Commonwealth of Independent States*
Armenia*
Azerbaijan*
Byelarus*
Georgia*
Kazakhstan*
Moldova*
Russia*
Ukraine*
Austria*
Belgium*
Finland*
France*
Germany*
Great Britain*
Greece*
Iceland*
Ireland*
Italy*
Netherlands*
Portugal*
Scandinavia*
Denmark*
Norway*
Sweden*

Spain*
Switzerland*
Vatican City*

North America*
Canada*
Alberta*
British Columbia*
Manitoba*
New Brunswick*
Newfoundland*
Northwest Territories*
Nova Scotia*
Ontario*
Prince Edward Island*
Quebec*
Saskatchewan*
Yukon Territory*

Caribbean Region*
Cuba*
Dominican Republic*
Haiti*
Puerto Rico*
Virgin Islands*

Central America*
Belize*
Costa Rica*
El Salvador*
Guatemala*
Honduras*
Nicaragua*
Panama*

Mexico*
Mexico City*

United States*
  Alabama*
  Alaska*
  Arizona*
  Arkansas*
  California*
    Los Angeles*
    Oakland
    San Francisco*
  Colorado*
  Connecticut*
  Delaware*
  District of Columbia*
  Florida*
    Fort Lauderdale
    Miami
  Georgia*
    Atlanta
  Hawaii*
  Idaho*
  Illinois*
    Chicago*
  Indiana*
  Iowa*
  Kansas*
  Kentucky*
  Louisiana*
  Maine*
  Maryland*
    Baltimore*
  Massachusetts*
    Boston*
  Michigan*
    Detroit

Minnesota*
Mississippi*
Missouri*
Montana*
Nebraska*
Nevada*
New Hampshire*
New Jersey*
    Newark
New Mexico*
New York*
    New York City*
North Carolina*
North Dakota*
Ohio*
Oklahoma*
Oregon*
Pennsylvania*
    Philadelphia*
Rhode Island*
South Carolina*
South Dakota*
Tennessee*
Texas*
    Houston
    Dallas
Utah*
Vermont*
Virginia*
Washington*
    Seattle
West Virginia*
Wisconsin*
Wyoming*

South America*
  Argentina*
  Bolivia*
  Brazil*
    Rio de Janiero
  Chile*
  Colombia*
  Ecuador*
  French Guiana*
  Guyana*
  Paraguay*
  Peru*
  Suriname*
  Uruguay*
  Venezuela*

Oceania

SN: Include here islands and island groups in the Pacific (e.g., Fiji).

At-Risk populations

SN: Being a member of an at-risk population does not put one at risk for infection. Risk behaviors that may be associated with these populations, not simply being a member of the population, are what put individuals at risk.

  Adolescents*
  Blood transfusion recipients
  Breast-fed infants
  Commercial sex workers
  Fetus*
  Firefighters
  Health care workers
  Hemophiliacs

Homeless persons*
Incarcerated persons

Law enforcement workers

SN: Include here all categories (e.g., correctional personnel).

Migrant workers>
Sexual partners of infected persons
Substance abusers
Tissue/organ transplant recipients (To include recipients of artificial insemination)

Religious Faiths

Buddhism*
Christianity*
  Eastern Orthodox
  Protestant
    Fundamentalism
  Roman Catholic>
Hinduism*
Islam*
Judaism*

Signs and Symptoms

Special Populations

SN: These terms are included because of their ubiquity in the epidemic. For condition or complication, SEE Stages of Infection.

Caregivers*
Discordant couples
HIV+ individuals
Worried well

Alphabetical Index

Pneumonia*, 42. *See also*
Pneumocystis carinii
pneumonia>; Bacterial
pneumonia>
Pneumonia, bacterial*. *See* Bacterial
pneumonia>
Pneumonia, pneumocystis carinii*.
See Pneumocystis carinii
pneumonia>
Pneumonia vaccine, 48
Podiatry*, 15
Poetry*, 70
Poetry therapy, 53
Pol>, 16
Polarity therapy. *See* Acupressure
Policies of AIDS service
organizations, 64
Policies of health care organizations,
64
Policies of private organizations, 65
Policies of World Health
Organization, 67
Political aspects, 62
Political parties, 63
Polymerase chain reaction*, 19
Polyproteins, 16. *See also* Proteins*
Polyradiculopathy, 44
Polyurethane condoms, 32
Poppers. *See* Etiology; Substance
abuse
Porphyria*, 42
Porphyria cutanea tarda*. *See*
Porphyria
Positive test, 18
Positron emission tomography>, 50
Post traumatic stress disorder>, 39
Posters, 69
Postsecondary schools, 30
Power of attorney, 61
Practice guideline*. *See* Practice
guidelines
Practice guidelines, 24
Pre-cum. *See* Pre-ejaculatory
secretions
Pre-ejaculatory secretions, 26

Pre-test, 18
Predictive value of tests*, 24
Pregnancy*, 29
Pregnancy complications*, 38
Pregnancy testing, 18
Pregnancy tests*. *See* Pregnancy
testing
Prejudice*, 63
Premarital testing, 18
Preschools, 30
Presumptive diagnosis, 46
Prevalence*, 25
Prevention, 27
Prevention and control*. *See*
Prevention; Universal
precautions*
Prevention of Infection, 47
Primary care, 48
Primary health care*. *See* Primary
care
Primary schools, 30
Princeton rub. *See* Frottage
Print sources, 19
Pro-gay, 63
Procedures (medical), 50
Procedures of AIDS service
organizations, 64
Procedures of health care
organizations, 64
Procedures of private organizations,
65
Proctitis*, 37
Proctocolitis*, 37
Proctology, 15
Products for safe, safer sex, 32
Professional issues, 56
Prognosis*, 46
Programs of AIDS service
organizations, 64
Programs of health care
organizations, 65
Programs of private organizations,
65
Programs of World Health
Organization, 67

Notes

For Product Safety Concerns and Information please contact our EU
representative GPSR@taylorandfrancis.com Taylor & Francis Verlag GmbH,
Kaufingerstraße 24, 80331 München, Germany

Batch number: 08153776

Printed by Printforce, the Netherlands